SUPERIOR SKIN

A Natural Way to Rejuvenate Your Skin

Find Out the Best Foods to Make Your Skin Fresh

Useful Tips and Simple Recipes

INTRODUCTION

The skin is the largest organ in the body, but unfortunately, it happens to be the most overlooked. Most of us think of the skin as that thing that covers our internal organs, and that's it. We don't think much about its essential complex functions; hence, we do not pay as much attention to our skin.

The best most of us do for the skin is we wash our bodies, with nice soap and water. We exfoliate occasionally, and that is just about it. The other part is not about care, even though most of us think it is; it's for our appearance, the tons of makeup (not limited to ladies by the way) we apply to enhance our looks – and most of the times covering up the effects of not properly taking care of our skin.

Does this sound like you? I believe you are here because you think that what you have been doing has not been working well, or for any other reason, you need to learn better ways to take care of your skin. The good news is that you came to the right place. This is not going to be another cosmetic tutorial, trying to sell you products laden with chemicals that may end up ruining your skin.

In this book, you will learn how to rejuvenate your skin, naturally, with natural products, and through what you eat, and yes, you can eat your way to rejuvenated, glowing skin. What foods, you may wonder? Well, I have not only given you food ideas but also included delicious recipes that you can try out immediately!

With this book by your side, you will know exactly how to improve your skin from the inside out and have glowing, even and beautiful skin.

Let us get started!

clarifying purposes only and are owned by the owners themselves, not affiliated with this document.

TABLE OF CONTENTS

Back to the Basics: Understanding Your Skin and Nutrients

While using the right products is important to the health of your skin, you also need to address your skin health from what you eat from the inside. Therefore, you have to use the inside-outside approach to improve your skin. In this chapter, we will focus on understanding the skin and how it works to understand better how to maintain its health.

Let us start by understanding the structure of the skin:

Structure of the Skin

The skin is made of 3 layers:

1. The Epidermis: This is the outer layer that we see and touch. It has four distinct layers, but it does not have blood vessels or nerve endings. It creates a waterproof barrier to the inner and more sensitive layers. Also, on this layer are melanocytes, which are special cells that produce the pigment melanin, which creates our skin tones (gives us color).

2. The Dermis: This is the middle layer. It is a bed of elastic connective tissue that provides strength, nourishes, and supports the epidermis. It also supports the nerve endings, blood vessels, sweat glands, lymph glands, and hair within it. It also contains fibroblasts and tissue microphages, cells that help to repair and protect the skin (the source of keratin).

3. The Subcutaneous Fat Layer: This acts as a shock absorber and protects the body from trauma. Otherwise known as the

hypodermis, this layer mostly made of fat and connective tissue helps the skin to attach to the underlying bone and muscle.

As you can see above, the skin is more than an outer cover for the body. The three layers perform the following functions:

- Regulation of body temperature

- Excretion, of toxins in the body as sweat through skin pores

- Protection: It protects the body from harsh environmental conditions.

- Sensitivity: It is the medium through which the body feels sensations such as warmth, itching, pain, or pressure.

- Moisture control: It keeps you from dehydration

- It is a large storeroom for the body, as the innermost layer can store fat, water, and metabolic products.

Essential Proteins for Skin Structure

There are three proteins in the skin that help maintain it in good condition. They include;

Elastin: This protein ensures the skin remains elastic; it allows it to stretch and spring back to its original position. Basically, it gives structure and support to the skin and organs. Elastin can be affected by factors such as time (age) and other elements such as weight gain. When overstretched, it breaks, resulting in silvery lines commonly referred to as stretch marks. When its production is diminished, the skin tends to wrinkle and sag.

Collagen: This is the most abundant protein in the skin, making up 75% of the organ. Found in the dermis, this is your fountain of youth; it is what wards off fine lines and wrinkles. The ability of the skin to produce this protein can be inhibited by certain environmental factors as well as aging. These factors can also break down existing collagen.

Keratin: This is the strongest of all proteins in the skin. It is responsible for ensuring the rigidity of the skin. It is also crucial for the growth and health of nails and hair.

Let us now look at the life cycle of your skin to understand this organ further:

The Life Cycle of Your Skin

The outer layer of the skin, the epidermis, is subject to renewal. A layer can last for up to 28 days, after which most of the cells are turned over and the most superficial ones replaced. Regeneration of new cells is much faster for infants, and it gets slower and slower as we age. For adults, it takes 28-42 days for the renewal to occur, while for people aged 50 and older, it could take up to 84 days.

The longer it takes the skin to repair and renew the old damaged cells, the more dead skin will be building up on your epidermis, which will make your complexion appear dull and your skin to look tired. It explains why we have skin that is more vibrant when we are younger, but this vibrancy may reduce as we age.

Factors that May Affect the Health of Your Skin

It is important to note that the skin is not only the largest organ but also one of the most responsive organs. It responds to many factors in your environment. The following factors will affect the health and appearance of your skin:

- Diet

- Stress

- Environment

- Climate

- Sun exposure

- Skin Products

Five of these factors are pretty obvious to most people, but we tend to ignore or downplay the first one; diet. At least many people know that a dirty and dusty environment and too much stress can affect their skin. We also know that some skin products can have adverse effects on the skin. However, most of us have failed to recognize the role diet plays in enabling you to have healthy skin. We do not think that what ends up in our stomachs will have any other effects on our appearance other than getting fat.

When we experience skin problems, the first stop is at the medicine cabinet and then straight to the 'natural cosmetics' that are easy to get these days. A turmeric cream, vitamin serums, charcoal mask, snail creams you name it – things we are convinced will solve our skin problems.

They work, sometimes, only that they are not permanent solutions. You may have to keep spending a lot of money on certain products to maintain healthy skin. However, it is essential to understand that you cannot solve a skin problem on the outside while it originates from the inside. Yes, you may mask it for a while, but you will have to address it from the inside to eliminate it for good and set your skin free.

The way to address skin problems from the inside is through nutrition. Therefore, you need to evaluate what you are feeding your body. Let's learn more about the connection between your diet and the health of your skin next.

Diet and Its Effect on the Skin

The health of your skin is greatly determined by what you eat. Unfortunately, many people spend tons of money getting creams, soaps, and other products with a promise to improve their skin.

You need to understand that healthy skin does not start with a particular special cosmetic product. Real healthy and beautiful skin begins with a healthy diet that promotes your general health, including that of your skin. Your skin needs to be nourished from the inside so that the same can be reflected on the outside. Well-nourished skin will be clear, supple, and glowing.

The right foods on your plate can give you that radiant and rejuvenated skin everybody wants – but very few get because they don't think food has got anything to do with it. It could be you are getting cosmetic treatments to ease your acne, but it is not getting better, and you wonder why. Did you know some foods trigger acne flare-ups?

This is why what you eat matters. Let us learn how some skin conditions are mainly brought about by your diet:

Acne

If you have recurring acne breakouts, the chances are that your diet is high in high-glycemic foods. These foods are easily converted into glucose in the body. Their effects on blood sugar and insulin lead to imbalances in hormones and other chemicals in the body.

For some people, this may lead to the skin reacting in acne flare-ups. No medicine or cosmetic applied would fix it. It would only correct the symptoms of the underlying problem. Therefore, unless you cut out the high glycemic foods, for instance, white flour, white rice, and eat whole foods instead, you will not be helping your skin to recover.

Eczema

This skin condition has been linked to diet. According to experts, food allergies can play a role in causing or worsening eczema. Therefore, you can adopt a suitable diet to manage this skin condition.

Dermatological experts advise that probiotics and probiotics found in food can help people suffering from eczema. Some foods that have naturally occurring bacteria include kimchi or kefir, a fermented dairy drink or live cultures such as yogurt. Probiotics are also found in certain types of dietary fiber, found in some vegetables, asparagus being a good source.

Good fats can also help with this condition; fats such as Omega-3. These fats help strengthen and improve the skin barrier function. Also, juice made from fruits and vegetables with anti-inflammatory properties such as beets, red grapes, black currants, cucumber, wheatgrass, celery, spinach, kale, zucchini and carrots can treat eczema.

Skin Aging and Sagging

Your skin can make you look tired and old with wrinkles and premature sagging even when you are not exactly old. The high glycemic diet that triggers acne is also said to fuel this. High glycemic foods can trigger glycation, non- enzymatic binding of sugar to proteins, which results in the formation of AGEs (advanced glycation end-products).

Glycation impacts protein molecules in the body and skin. Collagen and Elastin protein molecules in the skin become glycated when blood sugar levels are high – spiked by high glycemic foods. When they are glycated, they lose their mechanical properties and become dysfunctional. As discussed earlier, these molecules are responsible for keeping the skin tight, supple, and youthful. If they are dysfunctioning, the skin loses these 'aspects' which results in wrinkled, sagging, and old-looking skin.

Dry Skin

Are you experiencing cracked, scaly and dry skin, susceptible to breakouts and other infections? You might want to check your caffeine and alcohol intake. As natural diuretics, the more you drink alcohol and caffeine, the more dehydrated it makes you. They suck away your skin's natural moisture, leaving it dry and vulnerable. Before long, you may start to notice deep lines in your forehead, aging you before your time.

Sodium is yet another culprit responsible for dried-out skin. We consume sodium mostly in our table salt, used as seasoning to give taste to our foods. When we consume too much sodium, the body compensates by holding water, which not only leads to puffy cheeks but also cracked up and dry, dehydrated skin.

Oily Skin

Some of us have naturally oily skin, and the foods we are eating are not making it any better for us. If you find yourself dealing with clammy and sticky skin, sometimes causing acne breakouts, it could be you are consuming too much of the following; Dairy products, Trans fats found in most margarine, and deep-fried foods.

So what should you eat to have healthy glowing skin? Let us learn some of the best nutrients for great skin in the following chapter to help you know how to get started with improving the health of your skin.

NUTRIENTS FOR HEALTHY AND GLOWING SKIN

As mentioned earlier, the human skin requires nutrients to flourish. The skin is a reflection of what is happening inside your body. All your skin conditions, from acne to eczema or extra oily skin, are a manifestation of your body's internal needs, including nutritional needs. They tell you what your body has had enough of and what it needs. For instance, acne could be telling you, "Hey, I have had enough of this sugar. Give me some real, wholesome nutrients!"

If you feed your skin exactly what it needs and avoid things that harm it, you will have great skin, and will not struggle with some of the skin problems that you may be struggling with. You will not need to hide under caps and layers of makeup when you show up. Think about how easy it would be to wake up and show up without worrying about your skin, applying the makeup right to cover everything and worry about if it will stay put all day. If you are not worrying about your skin, imagine how free and confident you would be. Life is so much easier, better, and yes, cheaper with healthy skin from the inside out. However, it will come to you at a cost – a small cost to pay, given the benefits.

What is that cost? Feed your skin the nutrients for healthy skin while avoiding harmful substances.

So what are these nutrients that your skin needs for its optimal health, to feel and look its best? Let's find out below;

ANTIOXIDANTS

What are antioxidants? These chemicals protect the skin from damage by free radicals. When we talk about free radicals, we are referring to molecules with odd electrons that are highly reactive by nature. They are formed internally in our bodies during normal metabolism or by the immune system in its attempt to fight viruses and bacteria. Externally, they are formed as a byproduct of environmental factors such as sunlight, pollution, smoke, herbicides e.t.c.

As we age, it is easier for free radicals to damage our skin. As the skin ages, its main components oxidize because of the prolonged exposure to free radicals. Because they have lost an electron, these free radical molecules are busy in search of weaker cells in the body to take an electron from so they can complete themselves. When a healthy cell loses an electron, it becomes weak. When the cells are weakened, they become easy targets for bacteria and other factors that cause skin aging and damage. They may even end up dying. This is how free radicals damage and kill healthy cells, causing your skin to age and develop problems.

Antioxidants come in to protect cells from being damaged by these little nuisances called free radicals, which happen to be impossible to avoid. They neutralize the effects of environmental, metabolic, and immune factors that lead to the formation of free radicals. Antioxidants fight these damaging molecules; they engulf them, thereby counteracting their attacks, and then they eliminate them from the body.

What's more, antioxidants also strengthen cells, to build their resistance to free radical attacks on their electrons. More so for the skin, they play an essential role in protecting collagen and Elastin cells (we know how important for the skin these are, right?) from destruction.

Their protection of cell electrons helps prevent cell and tissue damage. Cell and tissue damage can lead to cellular damage and disease, leading to complicated skin conditions which sadly, we are out here trying to solve with 'special cosmetics' that cannot solve the problem at a cellular level.

But, how do antioxidants perform these protective functions?

They make the ultimate sacrifice of donating an electron to the desperate electron seeking free radical. Once it has the electron, it will not go harassing healthy cells, trying to steal one. The good thing is that antioxidants are pretty stable, and they do not become free radicals after donating an electron. They remain powerful enough to carry the free radicals with them as they are excreted out of the body.

Let us look at some of the most powerful antioxidants. We will start by looking at the vitamins that are antioxidants:

Vitamins

Vitamin C

This is the anti-aging superstar, with the following functions;

- It is crucial for the maintenance of the components that support the structure of the skin, namely Elastin and Collagen. It not only maintains collagen but also stimulates its production, to give your skin its firmness.

- It is the best for tackling wrinkles and dark marks, brightening dull skin such that it is visibly radiant and evening out uneven skin tone.

It is important to note that this antioxidant is notoriously unstable – especially in those bottled serums that are common nowadays. You could buy a nice one but then have it destroyed through exposure to light or air.

However, there is no such gamble with a diet rich in vitamin C, and you do not have to supplement it, as it is easy to get from your diet. You can find it in various fruits and vegetables that we shall discover below

Dietary sources of Vitamin C

Fruits

- Citric fruits, like the orange, lemon
- Pineapple
- Papaya
- Kiwi fruit
- Mango
- Cantaloupe
- Grape fruit
- Strawberries
- Guava
- Tomato

Vegetables

- Broccoli
- Brussel sprouts
- Cauliflower
- Sweet and white potatoes
- Hot green chili pepper

- Bell peppers

- Kale

- Spinach

- Parsley

Vitamin E

This vitamin is a soluble oil antioxidant playing the following roles;

- It helps protect the fat component of the skin from damage by free radicals.

- It also helps slow down the conversion of soluble collagen predominant in youthful skin to insoluble collagen associated with aging skin.

- It enables the skin to retain its moisture to soothe and moisturize dry or rough skin.

- Working together with Vitamin C, Vitamin E protects the skin from the damaging effect of Ultraviolet Rays (UV light). You are going to notice smooth skin if you eat foods high in vitamin E.

Dietary sources of vitamin E

Basically, vitamin E is found in plant-based oils, nuts, fruits, seeds, and vegetables. You can find it in;

- Almonds, Peanuts and Peanut butter

- Sunflower seeds

- Pumpkin

- Bell pepper

- Wheat germ oil, sunflower, soybean and safflower oil, and rice bran oil

- Avocado

- Mango

- Collard greens

- Spinach

- Beet greens (leaves of the plant bearing beetroot)

- Asparagus

- Butternut squash

- Trout

Vitamin B Complex

When we talk about vitamin B complex, we are referring to several various forms of Vitamin B, many of which play an essential role in the making of healthy skin. There is B-3, B-5, B-6 and Vitamin B-7, with the following functions;

- Vitamin B complex helps the skin to regulate cell-turnover and sebum production. It also helps it to use essential fatty acids efficiently.

- B-3 (Niacin), in particular, helps the skin to retain moisture so the skin can look plumper and younger. Its anti-inflammatory properties also help soothe dry and irritated skin.

- Of all these vitamin B forms, B-7, otherwise known as biotin, is the most important one found in the skin. Its deficiency may result in dermatitis, a skin condition characterized by itchy and scaly skin.

The body can make some biotin on its own. However, to get enough for the desired results, you should include foods rich in Biotin in your diet, as well as other Vitamin B forms.

Dietary sources of Vitamin B complex

- Salmon

- Leafy greens especially spinach, turnip greens, collards, and romaine lettuce

- Organ meats particularly liver

- Eggs (rich in B7)

- Milk (a good source of B12)

- Beef (contains high amounts of B3, B6, and B12)

- Chicken and turkey (high in B3 and B6)

- Yogurt (high in B12)

- Legumes such as black beans, green peas, roasted soy nuts and kidney beans (high in folate, a B vitamin)

- For those not interested in meat and eggs, consider eating vegetables, nuts, seeds, and whole grains, all of which contain small amounts of B7, Biotin.

Vitamin A

This is quite an essential nutrient for healthy, firm, and glowing skin. Vitamin A has incredible benefits for the skin;

- It protects the skin from photo damage resulting from prolonged exposure to ultraviolet rays of the sun. Photo damage is one of the leading causes of premature aging and cellulite as it affects the components that enable skin elasticity.

- Vitamin A promotes the growth of collagen, which helps keep the skin firm and also protects from sunburns, and it controls keratin production, the substance that makes up most of our skin cells.

- It suppresses oil glands and keeps them from producing excess oils, which in turn decreases the occurrence of acne.

- It helps with the regeneration of skin cells, which form the protective layers of the skin. These layers are responsible for protecting the skin against damage and skin conditions and diseases such as psoriasis, eczema, and dry skin.

Lack of vitamin A may lead to a dry and flaky complexion with old-looking skin. It also makes you prone to sunburns and skin diseases.

Dietary Sources of Vitamin A

- Pumpkin

- Sweet potato

- Leafy greens such as spinach

- Eggs

- Orange and yellowish fruits such as pawpaw, dried apricots, mango, cantaloupe melon tomatoes

- Fortified breakfast cereals

- Cod liver oil

- Beef liver

- Beta carotene sources such as carrot, broccoli

- Black eyes peas

- Goat cheese etc

Resveratrol

This is a potent polyphenol antioxidant compound with anti-inflammatory effects and also protects the skin from sun damage.

Dietary sources

- Red wine

- Grapes

- Cranberries and blueberries

- Nuts

Curcumin

Newly discovered, this antioxidant is believed to deliver anti-inflammatory and skin brightening effects.

Dietary source

- Turmeric

Notes on Consumption

- Leafy greens: They are among the best vegetable sources of folate B9 and almost all antioxidants. To get the most out of them, avoid cooking as they could overcook and lose essential nutrients – which can also transfer and be left in the cooking water. To minimize the loss of nutrients, steam the greens instead to be between tender and crisp.

- Organ meat: If you do not relish the taste of organ meat or you do not find them appetizing, try them ground and mixed with traditional cuts of ground meat.

- Eggs: They say you can get the most nutrients by eating some foods raw. This is true, but when it comes to eggs, this may not apply. This is one food you ought to eat cooked, and this is why: Raw egg whites contain avidin, a protein that binds with biotin (B7) and prevents its absorption in the gut. Cooking them inactivates avidin.

- Do not overcook anything, as too much heat kills nutrients. Also, find out which foods are best eaten raw and do just that (you do not have to cook everything).

Overall Benefits of Antioxidants

Generally, a diet rich in antioxidants, even those we may not have mentioned here will help your skin in these ways;

- Skin firming: they will reverse the effects of cell damage and aging to give you a firmer, youthful, and rejuvenated skin.

- Scar treatment: By accelerating the renewal of tissues, they can reduce the appearance of scar tissue. Usually, scar tissue has a different structure than that of healthy skin; it is rigid. What antioxidants, especially those found in aloe and allium extracts found in onions, do is that they increase blood flow to the scar tissue to minimize its appearance and blend it with the development of new skin.

- Repair of sun damage: Too much exposure to the sun can dry out and damage your cells, affecting both the health and appearance of your skin. Antioxidants help with the growth of new cells and rejuvenate sun-damaged skin.

- Reduce the appearance of wrinkles and fine lines: It may be impossible to make wrinkles disappear completely. However, with antioxidants, particularly vitamins C and E, you can make your skin plumper and reduce their appearance to get youthful skin.

- Anti-inflammation: By increasing circulation and cell metabolism, antioxidants can reduce inflammation, which helps keep acne at bay, kick wrinkles to the curb, and also to bring about more even skin tone.

Important to Note

Remember the adage that 'there is strength in numbers'? This is true, especially when it comes to the functioning of antioxidants; they work best together. Do not pick out one type to eat; combine several or all of them if possible. Create some colorful foods with various kinds of ingredients and reap all the benefits. By putting antioxidants to work together and combining them with other skin-beneficial ingredients, the results will be amazing such that you will be blown away.

Now that you know how important vitamins are not only for your skin but also for your general health, let us now look at

Minerals

We talk a lot about vitamins playing an essential role in our overall health, which they do. However, most of the time, we tend to overlook minerals, which, by the way, are very vital for general body and skin health. Minerals are so essential such that the vitamins would be useless if minerals did not compliment them.

There are about 16 minerals, which are known to be essential for human health. Most of these are only needed in trace amounts, which you can get the recommended dose in your diet. While they all contribute to the making of healthy skin, there are a few that are highly essential if you desire to have clear, glowing skin. Let's discuss them below;

Zinc

Zinc is the most important 'healing mineral' for the skin, especially useful for acne sufferers. Clogged pores caused by excess oil produced in the skin is the culprit in causing acne in many people. Zinc helps by controlling the amount of oil being produced in the skin and settling some hormones that can cause acne.

Zinc is also a wonder mineral that is believed to have antioxidant properties that protect against premature aging of the skin and the muscles underneath by attacking free radicals notorious for weakening cells as earlier discussed.

Also, in case your skin is injured, say scratched, or even after getting sunburned, the healing mineral reduces inflammation and helps your skin to heal and rejuvenate faster. What's more, zinc is known as a natural sunblock/sunscreen to protect your skin from harmful UV rays. Isn't it a wonderful mineral? So where can you get it?

Dietary sources of Zinc

- Animal protein (beef, pork, mutton)

- Seafood (lobsters, crab, oysters)

- Nuts (Brazil nuts, almonds, cashews, hazelnuts, walnuts)

- Sunflower seeds, sesame seeds

- Legumes

- Soy foods, fortified cereals

Note: It is crucial that you soak your grains, seeds, and nuts in water overnight before consuming them. This will help release the phytic acid they all contain, an acid that may interfere with the absorption of Zinc.

Silica

It sounds like silicone, and you are probably wondering how this can help your skin naturally, while you might have heard weird things about it and its use in plastic surgery. No, we are not talking about silicone; this is silica (which is not related to silicone), an excellent mineral for improving your skin, naturally.

How does it help the skin?

- Silica plays a crucial role in the production of collagen and glycosaminoglycans (GAGs), which helps in maintaining the skin's elasticity.

- It also helps maintain the body's connective tissues, muscles, cartilage and bone, tendons, etc., to keep them in place. This gives your skin form and shape; otherwise, everything would be hanging and skin sagging. This function also helps wounds to heal faster.

Silica deficiency can easily lead to losing skin elasticity, sagging skin, and slower healing of wounds. Combine it with Zinc for wonderful results. So, where can you find silica?

Dietary sources of silica

- Strawberries

- Mango

- Cucumber

- Celery

- Chickpeas

- Beans

- Leek

Selenium

Selenium is a strong antioxidant mineral fighting free radicals and essential in maintaining skin elasticity and flexibility. Also, this mineral is believed to have health benefits that could protect the skin from developing skin cancer as it also has properties that protect the skin from UV damage.

Selenium also improves blood flow, which is crucial for a healthy body and skin. It is also great at dealing with inflammation. So, which foods are high in selenium? Let us find out below:

Dietary sources of selenium

- Whole foods (rice, wheat e.tc)

- Sunflower seeds

- Brazil nuts

- Sardines

Calcium

We all know how important calcium is for the health of our bones and teeth, right? What most of us are not aware of is that calcium is also an essential mineral for skin health. So, how does it help the skin?

Calcium helps in maintaining the firmness and elasticity of the skin and other tissues and cells. It is also believed to be an acne-fighting mineral. There is no healthy body or skin without calcium as the human body contains and requires calcium more than any other mineral. If you lack enough calcium, your skin may become thin and fragile, and you may be more prone to acne.

Dietary sources of calcium

- Nuts (particularly hazelnuts, pistachios, and almonds)

- Leafy greens

- Dairy products (milk, cheese, yogurt etc.)

- Sesame seeds

- Collard

Note: Taking too much alcohol, coffee, and soft drinks, and too much stress can lead to calcium deficiency; it will break it down from your body.

Manganese

This is an essential mineral for the health of bones, hair, and muscles, and the skin. It is another warrior for fighting free radicals and supports the production of collagen. This helps keep the skin healthy and resilient. A deficiency of Manganese can lead to premature aging of the skin.

Dietary sources

You can get manganese from the following foods;

- Leafy greens (spinach, kale, collard greens)

- Oats

- Pumpkin seeds

Sulfur

This mineral makes up vital amino acids in the body, which help to maintain the structural integrity of our cells. Basically, it lives in our skin, bones, and muscles. Its deficiency would lead to wrinkles on the skin and muscle stiffness.

Dietary sources of sulfur

- Fish

- Brussels sprouts

- High-quality animal protein

- Eggs

Copper

You are probably wondering how the copper common to us as a metal can be eaten and benefit the skin. Well, relax; here we are talking about copper as a mineral, not a metal. Let me tell you how it benefits the skin;

It's quite the complimentary mineral, enabling others to work efficiently. Copper does help to enhance the function of antioxidants. Without it, they would not be as capable of fighting free radicals – it enables their efficiency. Also, copper foods are required to convert the amino acid tyrosine to promote hair and skin pigmentation.

Together with Zinc and vitamins, copper assists in the creation of Elastin, an element that keeps the skin flexible.

Dietary sources of copper

- Sunflower seeds, sesame seeds

- Brazil nuts, Hazelnuts, cashews, coconut

- Mushrooms

- Soybeans

Potassium

It is the regulatory mineral for the amount of water in your body's cells. Therefore, it helps the skin to stay hydrated, and a lack of it would probably lead to dry skin. Also, it is an electrolyte, holding an electric charge that is needed for cells to function normally

Dietary sources of potassium

- Lentils

- Kiwi fruit

- Bananas

- Oranges

- Milk

Note

As much as you ought to include minerals in your diet for your overall wellness, it is also important to eliminate foods that are going to deplete your mineral store. What good is it to strive to get minerals while you leak them out with foods you can avoid? Below are some foods that easily deplete your mineral stores;

- Trans-fats

- Alcohol

- Sugar and sugary drinks

- Processed foods

ESSENTIAL FATTY ACIDS

You have probably heard that fatty acids will keep your heart healthy. What you might not have heard is that these are one of those nutrient powerhouses that do not just target one part of your body, but instead, they work magic from head to toe. They benefit not only the inside of the body, but also their goodness will radiate on the skin.

So, which are these essential fatty acids?

There is a family of healthy fats referred to as omega fatty acids. There are 11 of them, but only two are considered essential fatty acids, as the body cannot make them on its own. They include Omega-3 and Omega-6. Of the omegas, the most critical for a healthy you are those two essential fatty acids and an additional one, Omega-9.

Let us learn how essential fatty acids are great:

The Beauty Benefits of Essential Fatty Acids

So, what do these wonderful fats do for your skin? They are the building blocks of healthy and vibrant, smooth, even, and youthful skin. This is how these essential fatty acids achieve that;

They keep the skin hydrated

The Omega-3s are a part of the skin's fat content. They boost the efficiency of its barrier function, which, if working correctly, acts as a seal for the skin; it keeps the moisture in and irritants and possible pollutants from the environment out. If the barrier is not working well, at times when the skin is compromised, say by exposure to harmful elements such as the sun, wind, or dust, its moisture escapes, leaving it dry, rough, and vulnerable.

Omega 3 fatty acids help to keep that seal strong, which keeps your skin moisturized, less rough, and less sensitive. What does this mean? There will probably be fewer breakouts if any because your skin is not easily irritated.

They protect your skin from harmful UV rays of the sun

We cannot help but be exposed to these harmful rays from time to time, and we must take steps to protect our skin from being damaged. Omega 3 fatty acids come in handy for this purpose.

Essential fatty acids have powerful anti-inflammatory effects. According to experts, these fats protect skin cells against inflammation caused by UV rays. They also regulate the body's response to those harmful rays, thereby mitigating damage.

When your body has been well nourished with these fatty acids, you do not have to worry much about those moments you find yourself outdoors. Your skin barrier is already equipped to fight off these rays.

They fight premature aging of the skin and wrinkles

We have many elements in our environment that won't just let our skin stay plump and youthful. They trigger inflammation and harm our collagen such that our skin does not remain tight, and bounce back when we make facial expressions, like creasing our forehead.

In due course, we might develop wrinkles around the eyes, the mouth, and on our foreheads. Without the support of skin structure by collagen, the skin may start to look loose and aged.

Omega 3, with its potent anti-inflammatory properties, helps fight any effects of factors that may cause inflammation. Also, it supports collagen, which in turn supports our skin structure, to keep the skin plump, reducing the appearance of wrinkles and keeping us looking younger.

A weapon against acne

We have already discussed vital nutrients to ward off acne, and essential fatty acids also make it to this list. This has a lot to do with their powerful anti-inflammatory properties since, according to experts; most acne may be primarily caused by inflammation, which is why Omega fatty acids have been found to fight acne.

So, what are great sources of fatty acids? Let's find out below;

Dietary Sources of Essential Fatty Acids

As mentioned earlier, they are referred to as essential fats because your body cannot produce them; you need to get them from an external source (your diet). The WHO (World Health Organization) recommends that we should eat foods rich in Omega 3 (oily fish) at least two times a week.

Remember, it's not just Omega 3 that is important; omega 6 and Omega 9 essential fatty acids are important too. The following foods are where you can get each group of fatty acids;

Omega-3

- Oily fish like salmon, mackerel, sardines, anchovies

- Chia seeds

- Flax seeds

- Walnuts

Omega-6

- Soybean oil

- Nuts (cashew nuts, walnuts)

- Sunflower seeds

- Corn oil

- Mayonnaise

Omega – 9

- Avocado oil

- Cashew nut oil, cashew nuts

- Olive oil

- Walnuts

- Almond oil

Note

These essential fatty acids are not to be taken anyhow, and not in excess – an excess is not good. You must be keen to strike a healthy balance between the essential oils consumed. For instance, the ratio between Omega -6 and Omega-3 ought to be less than 4:1.

Most people consume too much of omega-6s in their diet, while the body can produce omega 9s. However, most of us are not eating enough of Omega -3s. Therefore, in this case, the balance of the fatty acids is not near healthy – which is why we may not be enjoying all the benefits discussed earlier.

Oily fish two times a week and using olive oil in your cooking and salad dressings should give you a good balance of all those essential oils. Also, limit your intake of Omega- 6s by limiting the consumption of other vegetable oils and fried foods cooked in refined vegetable oils.

Bottom Line

As you can gather from our discussion above, there is more than one nutrient in some foods. For instance, leafy greens are a source of vitamins and minerals, too, therefore by eating them, you gain both ways. However, it is also important to note that there is nowhere where we have mentioned that high glycemic foods such as white rice, flour, cakes, fries, and such foods that we love eat contain any of these vital nutrients. Therefore, it has to be clear that a healthy diet, free from processed foods, high carbs, alcohol, and harmful fats (Trans -fats) is the key to healthy skin.

Now we know the types of foods we need to eat. There are nuts, vegetables, oily fish, whole grains, and healthy fruits. The question is, how do you pick out and combine the right ingredients to make a nutritious meal that is going to benefit your skin? You can be creative and mix them up according to your preferences, but if you are unable to do this, maybe because you are pressed for time, it is no reason to compromise your skin with the wrong 'quick' foods.

In the next part of this book, we are going to discuss diet plans for healthy skin. They involve all the healthy foods discussed and diet patterns recommended by experts to help in the development of clear and beautiful skin. These plans also include wonderful recipes for delicious meals that you can create in your kitchen, which makes it easier for you in so many ways.

For instance, you do not have to spend much time thinking about what to cook and what ingredients to choose. With a recipe, you know exactly what to buy in terms of ingredients (which make it easier to make a budget) and precisely what to cook and how long it is going to take. This will save you time, increase your efficiency, and make sure that you are eating right for your skin. Are you ready for this next part? Let's get started.

Diet Plans for Healthy Skin

In this chapter, we will look at various types of diets that incorporate some of those healthy nutrients we have mentioned that are good for the health of your skin:

The Mediterranean Diet

This diet reflects the traditional healthy eating habits of people from countries around the Mediterranean sea, which include Spain, Greece, Italy, and France.

The typical Mediterranean diet is characterized by a high intake of fresh fruit and vegetables, unsaturated fats like olive oil, whole grains, legumes, nuts, moderate consumption of fish and meat, and low consumption of sugar, processed foods, red meat, and dairy. It also allows for enjoyment of a glass of wine – in moderation.

You may probably be wondering what the Mediterranean diet has to do with your skin. As discussed earlier, high glycemic foods are bad for your skin healthy. They are the ones that will trigger inflammation, irritation, dryness, acne and other skin conditions. This diet removes high glycemic foods from your diet, getting rid of the 'irritants' which indeed helps your skin.

If you want to incorporate the Mediterranean diet into your lifestyle, here are some tips to guide you through;

- Eat healthy (unsaturated) fats: Olive oil is a suitable replacement oil tht you can use to cook intead of vegetable oil or butter. You could also use flavored olive oil on your bread in place of bread spreads such as margarine or butter.

- Use spices: Mediterranean dishes have plenty of natural spices. Not only does this make the foods a lot tastier but also, it reduces the need for salt, which will then reduce your sodium intake.

- More fresh fruits and vegetables: If you thought two slices of fruit is enough, think again. In this diet, you ought to aim for at least 7 to 10 servings a day of fruit and vegetables.

- Whole grains all the way: No more white bread or rice. In this diet, you have to switch from processed grains to whole grains. Therefore, buy more of whole-grain bread, brown rice, cereals, pasta, and other grains.

- More seafood: Fish twice a week is a must. Go for the following healthy types; salmon, tuna, mackerel, trout, and herring. You could cook them anyway you want to, but whatever you do, stay away from the deep-frying option.

- Reduce the consumption of red meat: Try as much as possible to reduce your intake of red meat, especially if it's fatty. If you eat red meat, get a lean piece, and keep your portions small. Otherwise, if you have to eat meat, go for the white meat substitutes such as chicken and fish – or go for beans.

- Some dairy is good, just not too much – and get healthy choices. Do not go for that attractive from the shelf sugary flavored yogurt. Instead, go for options such as low-fat Greek yogurt, plain yogurt, and cheeses, which are a much healthier option.

- Drink 6 to 8 glasses of water every day.

It is important to emphasize that this is not a restrictive diet, so if at all you eat plenty of foods high in sugar, salt or, fat,, your goal should be to reduce intake

Note

You do not have to get all of this right all at once or with every meal. Allow yourself to adjust gradually. Try to get it right for one meal, for a day, a week, and so on until it becomes a way of life. They say practice makes perfect – this is true, especially when it comes to switching up your diet or eating habits.

Mediterranean Diet Recipes

Are you wondering how to prepare Mediterranean-friendly recipes? We have got meal ideas for you. This section will provide you with recipes for breakfast, lunch, dinne, and snacks. Check them out and get started immediately as you learn to make more varieties in the future!

Breakfast Meal Ideas

Eggs and Vegetables

Ingredients

4 eggs, beaten

1 tablespoon of olive oil

2 minced garlic cloves

½ cup of arugula

1 cup of spinach

½ cup of shredded cheddar cheese

2 cups of steamed and chopped rainbow chard

Salt and black pepper to add some taste

Instructions

Set your heat to medium and heat the oil in a pan.

Fry chard, spinach, arugula for 3 minutes. Add in the garlic, stir and cook for more minutes.

Mix cheese and eggs then add into the chard mixture. Cook for about 5 to 7 minutes.

Season with salt and black pepper to taste.

Breakfast Pitas

Ingredients

2 sliced tomatoes

A handful coarsely chopped fresh parsley leaves

4 eggs at room temperature

½ cup hummus

2 cut in half whole wheat pita bread with pocket

1 cucumber, sliced thinly

Freshly ground black pepper

Hot sauce

Instructions

Cook the eggs in boiling water for 7 minutes.

Once ready, remove the egg and put it in cold water to cool. Peel it and cut into slices that are about ¼ inch thick, then sprinkle salt and put aside.

Spread pita pocket with hummus (about 2 tablespoons). Place the diced tomatoes and sliced cucumber in each pita. Tuck 2 sliced egg into each pita then sprinkle some salt

Serve.

Eggs Florentine

Ingredients

6 eggs, beaten

1 pinch of salt and ground black pepper

3 tablespoons cream cheese, sliced

½ cup of sliced mushrooms

½ package of fresh spinach

2 minced garlic cloves

2 tablespoons of olive oil

Instructions

Heat the oil in a pan over medium heat.

Add in the garlic and mushroom, and cook until they are soft, which should take about 2 minutes.

Add the spinach and cook for a few minutes.

Pour the eggs into the mixture and add salt and pepper for taste. Cook without stirring until the eggs are firm.

Sprinkle cheese over the mixture, cover for around five minutes or until the cheese melts.

Serve while warm.

Lunch Meal Ideas

Lemon Chicken Soup

Ingredients

1 sweet onion, sliced thinly

10 cups of chicken broth

8 minced garlic cloves

2 ounces crumbled feta

1 cup of pearl

3 tablespoons of olive oil

1/3 of chopped chives

½ teaspoon crushed red pepper

2 boneless/ skinless chicken breasts

Zest of 1 lemon

Salt and pepper

Instructions

Heat olive oil in a large 6-8 sauce pot at medium-low heat.

Once the oil is hot, add in the sliced onin and minced garlic. Cook until they are both softened.

Now add in chicken breast, crushed red pepper, lemon zest, and chicken broth. Cover with a lid and increase the heat to bring it to a oil.

Once boiling, lower the heat to medium-low and simmer for about 5 minutes.

Add in the salt and pepper to taste. Add in the couscous and cook on low heat for 5 minutes then turn off the heat.

Using a tong and a fork remove the chicken breast from the pot and shred the chicken using the fork.

Add the crumbled feta cheese and chopped chive into the pot. Add in the chicken and stir.

Serve warm and enjoy.

Grilled Chicken Kebab

Ingredients

1 teaspoon of kosher salt

1 small zucchini sliced into ¼ inch coins

½ teaspoon of freshly grounded black pepper

1 red bell pepper, cut into 1-inch pieces

1 kg of boneless skinless chicken breast

2 tablespoons dried oregano

¼ cup olive oil

1/3 cup plain Greek yogurt

4-5 cloves garlic pressed or minced

1 red onion quartered into 1-inch pieces

4 lemons juiced, plus zest from one of the lemons

Instructions

Slice the chicken into small pieces and place them in a bowl and set aside.

Mix the Greek yogurt and olive oil in a bowl. Add the lemon zest into this bowl. Add the lemon juice into the bowl with the yogurt. Add minced garlic, kosher salt, oregano, black pepper, and stir.

Pour half of the marinade into the bowl with chicken and reserve the rest for basting. Let the chicken marinate for about 3 hours in the refrigerator.

Prepare the grill by oiling the grate with some oil and cooking spray. Heat the grill to medium-high heat

If using metal skewers, no preparing but wooden skewers prepare them by soaking for 10 minutes.

Thread the chicken, red onion, zucchini, and red pepper on the skewer until the end of the skewer ending with chicken. Repeat with the remaining skewers, and then put the chicken on the grill.

Ensure you baste the kebabs with the reserved marinade, ensuring that you turn the skewers often to ensure each side turns brown and has light grill marks.

Cook until the chicken juice runs clear.

Serve while warm.

Shrimp Pasta with Red Pepper and Artichokes

Ingredients

1 cup canned artichokes hearts in water

3 minced garlic cloves

12 ounces of pasta

¼ cup of snipped fresh basil

¾ cup crumbled feta cheese, about 3 ounces

½ cup of dry white wine

¼ cup of butter

½ cup of whipping cream

2 ounces toasted pine nuts

1 ½ pounds of fresh shrimp on shells

2 tablespoons of lemon juice

3 tablespoons drained capers

1 ½ ounce jar of roasted red bell pepper drained and chopped

1 teaspoon finely shredded lemon zest

Instructions

Cook the pasta in a Dutch oven according to the instructions on the package, then drain. Return the pasta to the oven and cover to keep warm.

Melt the frozen shrimp, peel and devein shrimps, then rinse and dry them.

In a 12-inch skillet, melt the butter in medium-high heat.

Add garlic and shrimps, stir and let them cook for about 3 minutes.

Then add roasted pepper, wine, capers, and artichokes. Bring this to a boil, then lower the heat, simmer while uncovered until the shrimps are opaque.

Now stir in the whipping cream, lemon zest, and lemon juice.

Bring to a boil again, then boil gently while uncovered.

Into the cooked pasta, pour in the shrimp mixture and toss gently

Garnish with feta cheese, pine nuts, and basil.

Dinner Meal Ideas

Pork Chops with Sweet Onion

Ingredients

½ cup of water

1 teaspoon chopped fresh thyme

¾ teaspoon of kosher salt

¼ cup of raisins

1 tablespoon extra-virgin olive oil

I tablespoon of butter

½ teaspoon ground pepper

2 cups of thinly sliced sweet onions

½ cup of unsalted chicken broth

4 boneless pork loin chops about ½ inches thick trimmed

1 tablespoon of chopped flat-leaf parsley

3 tablespoons balsamic vinegar

Instructions

Heat oil in a large skillet.

Season the pork with some salt and pepper.

Once seasoned, put the pork into the skillet and cook while turning, until it browns each side. When ready, wrap the pork with foil then put it onto a plate.

Add onions and thyme into the pan and cook while stirring for 2 minutes. Now, add in broth and water and cook for 6 minutes ensuring that you stir often.

Stir in raisins and vinegar scraping up on any browned bits. Cook until it thickens

Remove from heat and stir in butter.

Serve the pork with the sauce topped with parsley.

Grilled Short Ribs and Tomatoes

Ingredients

1-pint cherry tomatoes

¾ teaspoon salt, divided

1 clove of garlic

1 tablespoon of lemon juice

1 pound of boneless short ribs or London broil

¼ teaspoon of crushed red pepper

1 cup of fresh parsley and cilantro leaves

2 tablespoons of red wine vinegar

½ teaspoon ground pepper, divided

2 tablespoons of extra virgin olive oil

Instructions

Preheat the grill at medium-high.

Season the mea with ½ teaspoon of salt and ¼ teaspoon pepper.

Grill the meat on a grill grate for 10-15 minutes making sure that you turn it occasionally.

Gill the tomatoes too and set aside one ready.

Place herbs, garlic, and remaining ¼teaspoon each salt and pepper in a food processor. Add oil lemon juice, vinegar, and crushed red pepper and process until the chimichurri is chunky and well-mixed

Serve the meat with chimichurri and tomatoes.

Vegetable Tagine

Ingredients

Juice of 1 lemon

1 tablespoon ground cinnamon

1 quart low-sodium vegetable broth (broth of your choice)

2 large russet potatoes, peeled and cubed

¼ cup extra virgin oil

1 tablespoon harissa spice blend

Handful fresh parsley leaves

Salt to taste

½ cup chopped dried apricot

10 chopped garlic cloves

1 large peeled and cubed sweet potato

2 cups of canned whole tomatoes

2 cups of cooked chickpeas

1 tablespoon ground coriander

2 large peeled and chopped carrots

2 peeled and chopped medium yellow onions

½ teaspoon of ground turmeric

Instructions

Heat olive oil in a large pot over medium heat until shimmering.

Add onion and increase the heat to medium-high, ensuring that you stir regularly.

Add all the chopped vegetables and sprinkle a little salt and spices. Then stir. Cook for 7 minutes while stirring.

Now add in apricot, tomatoes and the broth of your choice and cook for about 10 more minutes on medium-high heat.

Reduce the heat and cover then simmer for about 25 minutes until veggies are tender.

Add in the chickpeas and cook for another 5 minutes at low heat.

Now add in lemon juice and fresh parsley and stir. If you like, add harissa spice blend and a little salt.

Serve while hot with brown rice, favorite bread or couscous.

Keto Diet For Skin Health

The ketogenic diet, commonly known as the keto diet is a high fat, low carb diet. This diet has received a lot of attention on how it can promote weight loss and help manage cholesterol and blood sugar levels. However, there are suggestions that this diet can also promote healthy skin.

Caution

Some experts suggest that the keto diet has good and bad effects on your skin that you ought to know. However, if done correctly and with the right fats, this diet could be very beneficial for your skin.

The Proper Skin-Friendly Keto Diet

Carbs, usually the high glycemic ones, are linked to skin inflammation, which is a leading cause of skin condition as discussed earlier. The keto diet requires that you cut your carbohydrate consumption and eat more fats. The important thing is to know which carbohydrates you are cutting out, and which fats you are including in your diet.

For instance, by eliminating the simple carbohydrates high glycemic in nature, you help reduce inflammation in your body and skin. Without inflammation, your skin is going to feel more radiant, more open, and less congested or reddish.

When it comes to eating fats, you have to be very picky with what kind of fat you put on your plate and in what amounts. Choose healthy fat such as Omega3s and steer clear of Omega 6s. Again, you have to choose your sources of Omega 3 carefully.

Tips for a skin-friendly keto diet

- Your fat sources should be limited to Long-chain triglycerides (LCTs) such as; olive oil, avocado, soybean oil, nuts, fish, and white meats. Limit your intake of fat from MCTs (Medium-chain triglycerides), especially if combined with Omega fatty acids as they aggravate pre-existing inflammatory conditions like acne and psoriasis.

- Eat low carb veggies like cruciferous vegetables and leafy greens often. These help in hormone regulation and protect you from the side effects of glucose deficiency that you may suffer from when you go cold turkey on carbs.

- Limit or completely avoid dark chocolate as it may worsen acne.

- Limit or steer clear of dairy products. Dairy can sometimes increase the levels of insulin in the body.

- Do not take processed low carb foods. Instead, go for the fresh options. This is because foods such as processed meat do contain sugar, fillers, corn syrup, and other additives that could increase insulin levels and result in inflammation. If you cannot access fresh food, then please read labels to ascertain if what you are taking has no unwanted additives.

- Wait it out: It takes your body and skin a little while to adapt to this diet. Some people have reported worsening acne after switching to keto or any other low carb diet.

However, many have reported these 'side effects' to vanish after a short while, as it seems to be part of the keto-adaptation process. If you get such side effects, it could help to wait before you can reap the great benefits of skin-friendly keto.

Let us now learn how your skin will benefit when you adopt the keto diet:

How the Keto Diet Benefits the Skin

- The foods recommended for keto are high in antioxidants and low in sugar, which makes the diet an excellent anti-inflammatory diet.

- It has many offerings of high-quality fatty acids such as Omega 3, which are vital for skin health as previously discussed.

- The high oil content in the keto diet can be very beneficial for those with dry skin. More fat means more moisture and nourishment. As more oil is released onto the skin by the oil glands, your skin remains supple, giving it a dewy (glowing) and healthy appearance.

- High insulin levels stimulate the increased production of sebum and androgens, increasing the chances of developing acne. By limiting carbs, blood sugar is lower and a lot more stable and regulated, which, in turn, stabilizes insulin, the chemical that regulates the amount of glucose in the blood.

Keto Meal Plan for Clear Skin

Are you thinking how to mix up the right foods to make skin-friendly keto meals? Worry no more as we have some recipes that will ensure you prepare tasty keto meals every time, and you are going to love eating them as much as you are going to love your skin after you are keto-adapted.

Dinner/Lunch Meal Ideas

Salmon and Veggies

Ingredients

The salmon

2 salmon fillets at least 5-6 ounces each

Butter or avocado oil

Kosher salt

The kale

1 bunch black kale

2 cloves garlic – minced

Lemon zest and juice

Olive or avocado oil

½ cup red onion

¼ cup chicken stock/ or water

Black pepper and kosher salt

10 ounces baby bella mushrooms

¼ teaspoon red pepper flakes

The tomato salad

1 tablespoon extra virgin olive oil

2-3 radishes– thinly sliced

¼ teaspoon salt

A crack of pepper

1 1/2 cups cherry tomatoes - quartered

1 teaspoon parsley

Instructions

Making the salmon

It is important to dry out the skin, so that it becomes crispy and easy to remove. You can achieve this by putting the salmon in the fridge, skin side up for 30 minutes or even four hours. You then easily remove the skin.

Once the skin is out, set aside, then heat a non-stick pan over medium heat for around two minutes. Add two teaspoonful's of oil and wait for the oil to heat – 30 seconds should be enough.

As the oil heats up, season the salmon with salt on the part where you removed the skin. Place it on the heated oil, the skin side down. Season the top side with a pinch of salt and let the salmon cook for 5 minutes. If the edges on the top turn white or opaque, you know that the fish is ready to be flipped to cook on the other side. Flip the fish to cook the top-side. Lowe the heat a little bit to just below medium and allow it to cook for 5 minutes.

To know if it is cooked, squeeze the sides with your cooking spatula. If it feels firm, but with somewhat soft, then it is cooked. Remove from the pan and set aside on a flat dinner plate.

Preparing the kale

Separate the spongy part of the mushrooms from the stems and slice them thinly.

Remove stems from the kale and chop.

Place a large non-stick pan over medium-high heat. Add two teaspoonfuls of oil and let it heat up for 2 minutes. When the oil is hot, add the slices of mushroom and let them cook for 5 minutes. Once cooked, add the red onions, red pepper flakes, ¼ teaspoon of salt, and few cracks of pepper. Cook until the vegetables are soft.

Add in the garlic and then cook for one more minute. Add the chopped kale with an additional ¼ teaspoon salt. Pour in the chicken stock and cook until the kale is wilted (about 4 minutes).

Everything should be cooked by now. Turn off the heat and add one teaspoon lemon juice and the zest of half a lemon. Check the seasoning and adjust if necessary.

Preparing the tomato salad

Put the quartered tomatoes, parsley, and the sliced radishes into a bowl and mix them up. Add in the olive oil, salt, and pepper and mix again, but only when you are about to serve.

Serve the fish, with the kale and the salad on the side. Enjoy!

Sesame Chicken Thighs

Ingredients

7 ounces broccoli

3 tablespoons sesame seeds

1 lb chicken thigh with skin and bone

4 ounces almonds flour

2 eggs

Red pepper flakes (if you like)

3 ounces double cream

Salt and pepper to taste

For the garnish

 3 tablespoons spring onion

3 tablespoons low sodium soy sauce

2 tablespoons sesame oil

Lime juice

2 ounces thinly sliced bell peppers

Instructions

Preheat the oven to 400 F/ 200 F/ gas 6.

Take a large bowl and add the almond flour, sesame seeds, and sea salt. You can add in chili flakes if you like a little heat.

In another bowl, crack in the eggs, add the double cream, and whisk.

Dip the chicken thighs in the egg mixture, then dip in the sesame mix.

Line a baking sheet with parchment paper and place the chicken.

Cook in the oven for 30 minutes.

Steam or boil the broccoli until cooked but ensure that they are still firm. Place them in a bowl of cold water to keep them from cooking further.

The chicken thighs should be cooked after 30 minutes; remove them from the oven and drizzle on them the soy mixture and sesame oil.

It's time to serve! Serve the chicken with the steamed veggies. Make it even more colorful and delicious by sprinkling sliced red bell peppers and sliced spring onions. Serve with lime.

Keto Burrito Bowl

Ingredients

To make the cauliflower rice

2 medium-sized heads of cauliflower

1-2 tablespoons of chopped parsley

Grapeseed or avocado oil

2 cloves garlic – minced

Zest and juice of half a lime

½ red onion, chopped

Black pepper and kosher salt

¼ cup water or chicken stock

¼ teaspoon red pepper flakes

1 teaspoon each of smoked cumin, paprika and ancho chile powder

To make the pork chops

5 (5-ounces) boneless pork chops

Grapeseed or Avocado oil

1 teaspoon each of smoked paprika, cumin and ancho chile powder

Black pepper and kosher salt

To make the toppings

2 diced medium-sized tomatoes

Extra virgin olive oil

½ cup full fat shredded cheese (mozzarella, jack)

5 cups of finely sliced romaine lettuce

1-2 avocados

1 green bell pepper sliced

Black pepper and kosher salt

Instructions

Mix the paprika, ancho chile powder, and cumin in a bowl to make the spice rub for the pork chops.

Next, season the pork chops with salt and apply the spice rub evenly on both sides then drizzle 1 tablespoon of oil on each. Let them sit for 20-30 minutes at room temp.

Make the cauliflower rice by shredding the cauliflower heads with the largest setting on a boxer grater. Be careful to grate the florets, not too much of the stalks.

Heat a large pan with one tablespoon of oil over medium heat. Add the pepper flakes, salt, onions, and a couple of cracks of pepper and stir to mix. Cook for 5 minutes and add garlic, then allow it to cook for two more minutes.

Add paprika, cumin, and ancho and cook for a minute, stirring often. Add the chicken stock or water and stir to mix, and cook for 30 seconds before adding the cauliflower, a couple of cracks of pepper and ½ teaspoon of salt. Mix and cover the pan and allow to cook for about 4 minutes, stirring only once.

Taste the rice and, if cooked, turn off the heat. Add the lime zest, parsley, and lemon juice.

Cooking the chops

Heat a cast iron pan on medium heat for 2 minutes. Heat 1 tablespoon of oil for 20 seconds then add half the chops. Cook each side until a nice crust is formed and remove from the pan. Repeat for the other half of the chops.

Chop and prepare all the toppings and assemble your burrito bowl.

Serve! Top the cauliflower rice with the sliced chops. Enjoy!

Keto Smoothies For Glowing Skin

Below are low -carb green keto smoothie, which are healthy and without any added sugars:

Avocado Green Smoothie

Ingredients

½ cup almond milk

5-6 large mint leaves

¾ full fat coconut milk

3 sprigs of cilantro

1 teaspoon of vanilla

1 squeeze lime juice

½ avocado (4 ounces)

1 1/2 cups of crushed ice

Instructions

Other than the ice, place all the other ingredients in a blender. Blend on low speed until everything is completely pureed.

Add the crushed ice and blend.

*You can add an alternative low-carb sweetener for taste if you like it sweet.

Lemon Green smoothie

Ingredients

½ cup coconut cream/milk

3 tablespoons lemon juice

2 cups lightly steamed organic baby spinach leaves

½ large avocado

½ cucumber

1 scoop whey protein

1 cup of crushed ice

Xylitol or stevia to taste

Instructions

Get a high powered blender, and throw all the ingredients in. Blitz until evenly combined to get a smooth and creamy mixture. How thick do you love your smoothie? You could add water until you get the desired consistency (just not too much water that can 'drown' the taste).

Taste and adjust ingredients where necessary.

Serve! Pour into glasses; add your preferred toppings (it can be shredded coconut, organic blueberries, or 1-inch fresh ginger root, shredded).

Enjoy!

Strawberry Smoothie

Ingredients

2 tablespoons smooth almond butter

1 cup strawberries, frozen

1 cup unsweetened coconut milk

Instructions

Simply add all the ingredients to a blender.

Blend until smooth and to your preferred consistency.

Pour into a lovely glass.

Enjoy!

Breakfast Meal Ideas

Fried Eggs with Kale, and Bacon

This is perfect for breakfast. It will be ready in 20 minutes tops so you can get on with your busy day.

Ingredients

1 cup plain Greek yogurt

4 large eggs

5 tablespoons extra virgin oil – divided

4 slices bacon

½ teaspoon ground turmeric

1 bunch curly kale, remove stems and tear leaves into large pieces

Mild red pepper flakes and lime wedges (for serving)

Kosher salt

Instructions

Place a rack in the oven and preheat to 375 degrees.

Bake the bacon slices on a foil rimmed baking sheet until they turn brown. Tear them into large pieces and set aside the fat.

On another baking sheet, spread out the kale and drizzle with two tablespoons oil. Massage the oil into the leaves, season with salt, and bake for 5-7 minutes until lightly browned on the edges.

Season the yogurt with a pinch of salt and divide among the plates (4 servings) and top with bacon and kale.

Use a large non-stick skillet to heat the remaining 3 tablespoons of oil over medium-high heat. Break in one egg at a time, shaking the skillet once at a time to keep the eggs from sticking together.

While cooking, tilt the skillet towards you, spooning the egg whites over so that they are set. Cook them for about two minutes.

Divide the eggs among the plates and enjoy. You could sprinkle the red pepper flakes and squeeze the limes onto them for that zesty taste.

Enjoy!

Intermittent Fasting for Healthy Skin

Intermittent fasting (IF) is more of an eating pattern than a diet. While practicing IF, you eat during a particular window known as the eating window, and for the rest of the time, the fasting period; you consume zero calorie foods or nothing, or you eat limited calories.

IF is known to contribute to weight loss, building of lean muscles and a stronger immune system. A little known benefit of this eating pattern is that it helps revitalize your skin through detoxification – and autophagy.

How Cell Detoxification and Autophagy Works

Autophagy literally means 'self-eating.' It is an evolutionary process of cells, whereby the body recycles cells by targeting the damaged and dysfunctional cells. It digests them and creates new healthier cells. This process refreshes the skin, and this helps it in so many ways. The autophagy process is accelerated during times when our body is experiencing certain types of stress, such as when we skip meals and consume lesser calories than needed.

According to experts, skin aging is can sometimes be caused by defective autophagy. This is because the cellular process that causes aging is increased by the presence of damaged molecules (cells) within cells that would have been consumed if there was effective autophagy.

It does not just protect the skin against aging; autophagy also protects the skin from infections and skin conditions such as acne, vitiligo, and psoriasis. It achieves this by preventing inflammation, reducing oxidative stress by free radicals, and maintaining the skin barrier function.

The calorie restriction in IF is not just for weight loss; it also increases your stem cells, which in turn boost cell growth and tissue homeostasis, also a part of the autophagy process.

Let us now learn how to practice intermittent fasting for better skin:

How to Practice Intermittent Fasting

It is not a one size fits all kind of diet pattern. There are several versions of IF of which you can choose the one best suitable for you depending on your gender and, most importantly schedule. The most common versions include;

- The lean gains protocol (16:8) – You have an 8-hour feeding window and 16 hours fasting period.

- The warrior diet (20:4) – You get 4 hours feeding window and 20 hours fasting period, but you can eat low-calorie healthy snacks in between.

- 5:2 diet pattern, which involves five days of eating as you normally do and two alternate days of zero calories.

Choose an intermittent fasting method that fits you. Do you think that going 16 hours without food is not doable, then opt for something else. Also, the good thing is, you can schedule your fasted period to be during your sleeping hours to make it easier to stick to the plan. At first, you may struggle with hunger, but after a while, you will not be as hungry every 2 hours.

Now that we have learned about various diet plans you can adopt for healthy skin, let us now look at how best to prepare your food to yield the most health benefits.

How to Get the Most Nutrients out of Your Food

Most of the time, we get the right foods with the right nutrients from the grocery store or whatever food store. Unfortunately, very few of those nutrients do end up in our bodies. Why is that? We eat them in the wrong form, cook them wrong, or fail to pair them with the right foods.

Below are essential tips that will ensure that you get the most nutrients out of your food.

Eat Raw or Cooked?

It is crucial to find out which foods are best raw and which ones are better off cooked.

- Eating raw and less processed foods may not be the best option for some foods. For instance, canned tomato products have four times more lycopene than fresh ones. Eating cooked eggs is also better than eating them raw, as we mentioned earlier in the book.

- Be careful when cooking foods rich in water-soluble vitamins like Vitamin C and B complex, foods like asparagus, winter squash, leafy greens, and beans. With such foods, cook them in low heat and use little water to prevent loss of nutrients through overcooking (too much heat) or by them dissolving in the water. Also, use any leftover cooking water to make soup as it contains vitamins that leached from the food.

Be mindful of how you prepare some foods as it can make all the difference in the vitamins, minerals and other nutritious compounds you get to access. You may not think this is important but the basics of food preparation such as chopping, crushing, soaking and blending make a huge difference.

For instance:

- Crushing and chopping garlic and onions releases aliinase, an enzyme that helps form a nutrient, allicin, the important nutrient in these foods.

- Cutting vegetable and fruits breaks down rigid plant cell walls, releasing locked in nutrients.

Proper Pairing

Pairing or rather eating some foods together facilitates the absorption of some nutrients. For example;

- It would be beneficial to pair fatty foods with foods rich in fat-soluble vitamins like Vitamins A, E, D, and K and also some antioxidants like lycopene. For instance, the fats in olive oil will help in the absorption of beta-carotene in your red peppers or oranges. Therefore sprinkling it in your food will be beneficial.

- It will help to get the best of calcium by combining foods rich in Vitamin D with calcium-rich foods, as this helps with calcium absorption. Therefore, have your vitamin D rich foods such as eggs or salmon with a calcium source such as yogurt or milk.

- Pair iron and zinc with foods rich in sulfur as the sulfur mineral binds to these minerals and betters their absorption. For instance, foods like beef and turkey rich in zinc and iron go better with garlic and onions, usually rich in sulfur.

Eat Fresh and Local

If you can access locally grown foods, such as beets, carrots, or leafy greens, ensure that you eat them as soon as they are picked, fresh from the farm quite literally, as this maximizes the amount of nutrients you get from these foods. According to experts, the longer produce is removed from its source of nutrients (mother plant), the less nutritious it gets.

Eat the Rainbow

Mix things up, fruits, vegetables, and everything else to make a rainbow on your plate. Did you know that the color in vegetables and fruits come from vitamins and phytonutrients, the naturally occurring micro-nutrients? By making a rainbow on your plate, you will be getting more nutrients all at once.

Check your Tolerance

Even if a food is nutritious, it will not do you any good if you have an undetected food tolerance that keeps you from absorbing it. If you get bloating or problems with your stool after eating certain foods, consider an elimination diet. If you do not tolerate certain foods, for example when they are raw, you are better off avoiding them.

CONCLUSION

Thank you again for reading this book.

I hope that you have learned the most beneficial foods to eat to improve the health of your skin. Thus, before you go buying cosmetics to revitalize your skin, buy the right foods to enrich your skin from the inside out. Eat healthy foods, in the right forms and combinations and get the best of their nutrients.

Finally, if you found the book valuable, can you recommend it to others? One way to do that is to post a review on Amazon.

Please leave a review for this book on Amazon by visiting the page below:

https://amzn.to/2VMR5qr

Thank you, and good luck!

If you enjoyed this book, check out more books by Ambrose Kane

https://www.ambrosebooks.com/books